Bone Broth Power:

Reverse Grey Hair and Bring Back Morning Wood

Copyright © 2015 Greg Cleland

All rights reserved. No part of this publication may be reproduced, stored in a retrieval system, or transmitted, in any form or in any means - by electronic, mechanical, photocopying, recording or otherwise – without prior written permission.

Table of Contents

1. Introduction — 1
2. What Is Bone Broth and Why Is This Food Amazing? — 5
3. What Materials and Tools Do You Need When Preparing Bone Broth? — 12
4. The Best Bone Broth Recipes — 20
5. Is Bone Broth a Magic Potion for Your Health? The Great Benefits of Bone Broth — 29
6. Bonus Tips and Tricks — 40
7. How to Add Flavor to Your Bone Broth — 44
8. Conclusions — 47

1. Introduction

We often forget the value of food we may consider to be bland, old-fashioned, or not tasty enough. However the most precious treasures are frequently hidden beneath an appearance of commonality. There is a reverse to the well-known saying that not all that glitters is gold: not everything that seems modest or boring is worthless. There's a lot of wisdom in the famous lines from Tolkien: "a box without hinges, key, or lid, yet golden treasure inside it hid." Some of the most valuable things come with a dull or opaque surface and only after we get to know them closely do we realize what benefits they conceal.

So what about reversing grey hair and bringing back morning wood? Is this book a fantasy novel about the Holy Grail? Although you won't read fiction or allegory in the following pages, it would be fair enough to say this book is indeed the key to a source of power many of us are not familiar with. Through its innumerable benefits bone broth can truly be considered to be a potent catalyst for better health, rejuvenation, and vigor. By incorporating this magic food in your regular diet and consuming it on a daily basis in high quantities, you will certainly notice how your body gets its energy back and how you are actually able to slow down aging processes.

The key to taking advantage of the multifaceted benefits of bone broth is having faith in a holistic approach to your health. You may not spot highly evident effects right away; however if you consume bone broth regularly, you will sense your overall state improves and your energy levels are higher. This way you will actually play a trick on your biological age only by means of a type of food that is incredibly inexpensive, easy to prepare, and versatile. Now you don't have to empty your wallet each time you try out something that can keep you young and healthy for a longer time. Coenzyme Q10 or Viagra are not exactly cheap, are they? Well, all you have to do is turn bone broth into one of the basic parts of your diet and you'll notice you feel brighter and invigorated in the morning to your own joy and to the pleasure of anyone close to you.

Bone broth is a type of precious food that many of us don't know enough about. It seems so simple, even a bit crude! It doesn't look like any delicatessen, it's not very modern, and apparently it's made of "remains" from other dishes we often enjoy. How could it be worthy of our attention? And yet the marrow of the bones we consider to be so trivial is extremely rich in nourishing substances that our body is in great need of. Even though we may think bone broth tastes "ok" rather than "amazingly delicious", this book is your guide to discovering the numerous benefits and charms of this food. Not only will this book show you how helpful for your health bone broth can be and what amazing properties it actually has, but also it will inform you about the best methods to prepare bone broth. After you read this book, you'll have all it takes to incorporate it in your routine as a tasty food. In this book you will find a few great recipes and the best tips to cooking bone broth in a way that will make you love it. You don't have to consume it only as a necessary ingredient in your menu. Besides, you will also be informed about the tools and materials you will need for preparing awesome bone broth. Yes, you can teach your whole family about the health benefits of this food and you can cook great dishes for all of them!

Many of us probably only eat bone broth when we have to diversify our food. Maybe our grandmother used to prepare bone broth sometimes and we recall the taste, that's why from time to time we let ourselves cook it out of nostalgia or because we don't have something we deem more sophisticated at hand. Honestly, how many times per month do you cook bone broth? Or should we ask how many times per year? We live in a time when the market offers us so many options when it comes to food, that all we need is plenty of money in order to satisfy all our cravings for everything we see. We often go for exotic food in our attempt to experiment and explore many different cuisines and cultures. Sometimes we even "compete" with our family or friends when it comes to the food we cook and eat: who is a more ingenious cook? Who found something unique and barely discovered this weekend to share with the rest and even slightly boast about it? Although you may not do it in a conscious, deliberate, or regular way, you have certainly behaved like that at least a few times. Some of us are more careful about our health and may not be such gourmands. However even in that case bone broth is the last food we think about. If we want to eat healthy, we choose organic food or we go vegan. When we also want to lose weight, we prefer the paleo diet or we go on a juice detox, just because they are so modern and we've heard that many people follow them. That's our way of staying "in-style" when it comes to health and nutrition trends. And yet we often overlook such a nourishing food as bone broth for which you don't necessarily need a whole diet or nutrition program: you can savor it as such, just by incorporating it in your normal menu and routines. Read on and discover the reasons why you should start consuming bone broth and enjoying its benefits right away!

2. What Is Bone Broth and Why Is This Food Amazing?

First of all you should know that some ardent "admirers" of bone broth who have discovered its hidden treasures and have consistently included it in their regular food have done it through adopting a broader frame, the paleo diet. Why? Because it fits its basic principles so well and some people discovered it can perfectly be used as a staple for this diet. However regardless of the frame you want to choose for your bone broth (whether you need to make it part of a more complex program or not), you will certainly ensure that your overall health improves by means of consuming this food.

It would not be far-fetched to say bone broth is like a magic potion for your body. Is that even possible for such a seemingly mundane food? You're probably tempted to think even bread is more special than bone broth. What is bone broth after all? Isn't it that food your grandparents ate on their "darker" days? Isn't it kind of rural or old-fashioned? Isn't it "lower class"? Isn't bone broth just some water and bones boiling together to appease someone's hunger when that person lacks something more appetizing and consistent in their home ... the kind of food you prepare in a hurry, after you buy some bones from the market next to your house, because you don't have time or money for something more cool?

Actually no, bone broth is a wonder food. You will think: "Wait! I thought bone broth is kind of gross and useless." Don't you just buy some bones if you're out of money for real meat? Don't you just eat (or drink) that liquid in order to fill your stomach with something – anything? When there are so many vital nutrients in meat, vegetables, or legumes, how could bone broth even satiate you, let alone nourish your body? Well, we forget that bones contain lots of minerals and their marrow is highly concentrated. Some people consider chicken soup to be the all-inclusive healing liquid food, the "natural penicillin". Do you remember when your grandmother or your mom prepared hot chicken soup to keep a cold away or just to "feed your soul"? Most probably you do, don't we all? Only the thought of it made you feel better or warm inside and nobody can complain a well-prepared chicken soup is not delicious. However nobody knows that bone broth is actually much more nourishing. It can keep illness away from your body in many complex ways and it can make you feel energized and youthful. It's not only something you eat to warm up your flesh and spirit.

There are some preconceptions regarding bone broth, as you could see. Now let's clarify what exactly bone broth is for those of you who may not be familiar with all the details. This food is highly appreciated in Asia (where especially beef bone broth, fish stock, and fish bones broth are widely consumed) as well as in Europe. However in Europe more emphasis falls on stock and broth generally rather than on bone broth. What is the difference? All these types of food are prepared in quite a similar way by means of animal ingredients. In all of them you boil everything in water and you add vegetables and spices for taste. After you place the meat and/or bones in water, you skim the liquid and in the end you separate the meat from the bones. Eventually you keep only the liquid by straining the broth or stock through a fine sieve.

Stock is typically made of bones that also have some amount of meat left. They have to be boiled for 3-4 hours till the nourishing substances (as well as the taste) are transferred into the water and you can consume both the pieces of meat on the bones and the liquid thus obtained. Sometimes the bones are roasted so as to ensure a better taste. Broth is made of meat which sometimes includes smaller amounts of bones. Its preparation time is much shorter (about one hour for chicken, for instance). However there are people who consider stock to be a thinner version of broth – what remains after you sieve your broth. Others claim that broth is actually seasoned stock. If there are disagreements about the exact difference between broth and stock, everyone seems to have the same opinion when it comes to soup. This food is definitely a top dish in everyone's eating routines. Soup often uses broth as a basis for a more complex preparation: you place several other ingredients in your broth e.g. meat, vegetables, beans, grains etc. Soup is the conventional dish made through boiling meat (or bones) that is served in most countries all around the world with certain variations on the same theme, of course. Soup is the totally "noble" counterpart of stock or broth and everyone already consumes it.

What makes bone broth special in this case? Why is it different from stock? Bone broth implies using the same kind of ingredients, but the cooking time is much longer (it can even amount to 24 hours). Unlike stock, bone broth is consumed especially for its concentrated nutrients. It's not only prepared and used for its high amount of gelatin. Similarly, bones should be roasted for the bone broth if you want an exquisite taste. What is your sign that your bone broth is ready? If you can press the bones and they are soft or if the bones crumble when pressed between your thumb and your forefinger, then you can consider your bone broth ready.

"All right," you may think. So why should you spend so much time boiling bones when hardly any real food comes out of it? Why not cook roast chicken and chips or salmon instead? Is anyone trying to kid you into softening bones for hours in a row for nothing? The answer is no. Absolutely not. Bone broth is an incredibly rich source of proteins and minerals, an all in one type of food. You don't have to mix a dozen ingredients to get them all together for a meal or buy expensive supplements anymore. You can consume bone broth on a regular basis! What does that mean exactly? Well, you should know there are people who have discovered the particularly healing and nourishing effects of this food and consequently they consume bone broth every day. It's part of their daily menu not only during meals, when they try to eat it instead of the more common soup, but also between meals. If you usually drink tea or mineral water between meals, now you can reduce their quantity a bit and replace them with bone broth. It will definitely be more powerful for your organism!

Bone broth is incredibly easy to prepare, although it may seem you have to cook it for a long time. You don't actually have to be there and stir the pot continuously. Bone broth contains a lot of glycine, a substance that supports the detoxification processes in our whole body and it is used in the synthesis of hemoglobin or bile salts. Most processes involved in digestion are facilitated through the presence of glycine. It helps considerably with the secretion of gastric acids. Another precious component of bone broth is proline which supports the health of our skin. Gelatin is also amazing for our digestion.

Who should consume bone broth? Basically it's great treatment for anyone who wants to feel more healthy and energized through the day. It is especially recommended to those who feel weak or are sick (e.g. they suffer from chronic fatigue or depression). It is like a real potion for people whose immune system needs improvement. As already emphasized, it regulates digestion and metabolism. You should also drink bone broth to keep yourself hydrated. Drink plenty of broth during a day; drink it instead of 4-5 glasses of water! Bone broth also regulates your appetite. If you tend to feel too little hunger for some reason, it will stimulate you to eat. If you are prone to eating too much and in a chaotic way, bone broth is your cure. It will literally feed your body with many nutrients while making you feel less hunger when you shouldn't crave food. If you suffer from upper respiratory infections or you are sensitive to flu and colds, you should definitely include bone broth in your menu. Overall anyone who wants to feel stronger and more optimistic is also welcome to try out this amazing food and boost their energy levels and their mood. If you have problems with your bones or teeth …it is only natural to consume bone broth. Numerous substances that could be insufficient in your body and the reason why you're having problems can be solved by means of this magic food.

Last, but not least, if you (feel) you are growing older and you don't have as much sexual prowess as in your youth, start playing a trick on time by means of consuming bone broth. This is your weapon against the passage of time that may have been too unexpected or too quick. Start eating bone broth right after reading this book, don't hesitate and don't delay taking action for the improvement of your energy and your health!

3. What Materials and Tools Do You Need When Preparing Bone Broth?

You should keep in mind that bone broth is one of the least expensive types of food you can include in your menu. Once you understand it is not actually "cheap" (as in "having little value") you will have absolutely no more preconceptions regarding this wonderful food. Why do you think only expensive food is worth eating? If you go for the taste as a priority, sure, without any doubt, many things that are delicious also cost some good money. However bone broth is primarily valuable through its high content of minerals, vitamins, and proteins. You can add ingredients to make it taste great once you decide to make it part of your routine.

Your typical material for bone broth includes bones, vegetables, herbs, optionally meat, some form of acid, and lots of pure cold water. What kind of bones should you use? The most common types of bone broth are made of chicken, beef, and even lamb ... strange as it may sound to some people in various parts of the world who are less accustomed to consume this kind of meat. However don't limit yourself to these "classic" bones for broth. Choose what you prefer out of a larger list: chicken, beef, pork, lamb, fish, turkey, veal. Just go to the butcher's and choose whichever bones you want. Experiment with several bone types and decide what your favorite flavor is. Chicken, beef, turkey, and fish are very rich in nutrients and quite easy to find. Veal and lamb may be more of a rarity – but still you can track down your own supermarket or butcher's where you can trust you'll find them. For many people chicken, turkey, and beef seem to be the most versatile and "eater-friendly" in terms of taste. Anyway don't let yourself be influenced by convention or by other people's habits. Just try out several types of bones for your broth and decide on a few you want to consume regularly.

The best bones for broth are knuckle bones and feet (thanks to their large quantities of gelatin) as well as marrow bones (for their minerals and other nutrients). Marrow bones are also quite interesting for the taste – marrow adds a distinct flavor to the whole broth. For a bit of color and extra flavor, add meaty ribs and neck bones. Most people prefer roasting the bones before boiling and skimming them. We definitely agree with this general opinion. However should you like your bones as you buy them, don't hesitate to cook them your own way. Just cooking your bones slowly will already impart a lot of flavor to your broth. If you want to prepare a special kind of bone broth, the so-called "brown" variants, you will have to roast the bones.

Adding meat to the broth is a good idea, although rest assured you can also cook your broth with bones and vegetables only. However for extra proteins and taste, it is quite recommended to use some meat leftovers, too: for instance, some chicken carcass that you don't need for another dish or some pieces of meat that remained from your recent dishes. Alternatively you could even use large pieces of meat or a whole chicken. However you do want your broth to taste like bones and be special. For your health improvement purposes only bones and a few extra small pieces of meat are enough. You should not leave the meat in your broth longer than the normal time you usually need for cooking meat. After they boil together, remove the meat and leave only the bones to boil further. Ideally you should use fresh meat instead of frozen. Besides, meat from certain body parts is better, given its high concentration of collagen. Use mainly meat from the shoulder or shin area which is rich in connective tissue. It goes without saying that you should use high quality meat for your broth. If you can afford organic meat or meat from grass-fed animals, it is great. Otherwise you can buy your regular meat, just make sure it's not the lowest quality on the market.

You should add vegetables for their large amount of vitamins, because your aim is using broth for energizing and rejuvenating purposes. Of course they are not mandatory, but vegetables are not very expensive and you can surely find a few to enrich your broth with nutrients. You can use basically anything you like: carrots, celery, tomatoes, potatoes, turnips, etc. What you should keep in mind is that cabbage, broccoli, or cauliflower are not the best choices, given their high quantity of sulfur. They will change the taste of your broth a bit and you don't want it to be bitter. Add vegetables towards the end of the cooking, as that will preserve minerals and vitamins in a more pure form in the broth. You can add your favorite spices: dill, parsley, bay leaves, basil, estragon, rosemary etc. One tip to remember is that they can be removed easier in the end if you place them all in a sachet. Add as many spices as you want!

An essential element you need for bone broth is acid. Why is it so important to boil the bones in water that contains acid? There is a very scientifically sound reason for this: since bones contain lots of minerals, boiling bones in water somewhat resembles the human digestion. Cindy Micleau, a specialist in the benefits of this food for health, explains how hydrochloric acid breaks down the food into nutrients during our digestion and helps with the extraction of minerals from food. A similar process takes place when you cook bone broth and for this reason you need to pour some acid e.g. apple cider vinegar in your bone broth water, if you really want to make the most of the nourishing qualities of this food. What if you don't like the taste of vinegar, whether apple cider or balsamic? That will be absolutely no problem, because you can be pretty creative with your bone broth, as long as you add acid. You can use wine or lemon juice. Please keep in mind that adding acid to your broth will also improve its taste considerably and you'll enjoy consuming your healing medicine for pleasure.

Some of you may already know it is best to use cold water for your broth. Why? It all comes down to the chemical processes that take place during boiling: if you place the meat, bones, or other ingredients directly in pure cold water, you will make sure their fibers will open gradually and their juices will be released slowly. It is best to let the bones warm in water in the most natural way rather than "throwing" them in already hot water. One extra tip for keeping all the nutrients intact is soaking the bones in cold water in which you also added vinegar (or another acid). If you leave the bones for your broth for about one hour in cold water in which you added vinegar and only afterwards get them to boiling, your both will be as nourishing and as tasty as it gets.

There are also other ingredients you can freely add to your bone broth to improve its taste and quantity of nutrients. We will list them all in a following chapter. At this point you know the basics about what materials you need to prepare bone broth that is good enough. Anything you can and may want to add to your bone broth "melting pot" is already a rather creative act about which you'll find out more tips a bit later.

If you ask yourself whether you'll have to spend half of your monthly salary to purchase special kitchen tools and supplies once you start going on a so-called bone broth health program, the answer is negative. Don't worry, you don't actually have to chop the bones yourself! Ideally you should just find a great butcher's store and bring everything home in the form that you will prepare it. You won't need much more apart from your classic cook's knife to chop vegetables. As for the pot that you should use for cooking bone broth, it should be made of stainless steel. You need a pot that is large enough. It should let you comfortably boil about 5 gallons of liquid. Since some of the bones may be a bit larger (e.g. backbones, legs, ribs etc.), you should make sure there is enough space for everything. Remember you'll also have to pour plenty of water, so make sure you don't just press and squeeze your bones and vegetables into any pot you have at hand in your home. Ideally you should save a large pot just for bone broth or purchase a new one for this purpose. It's not something that's expensive and it will definitely be worth the money, given all the health benefits you'll get! You can comfortably use a crock pot or slow cooker.

All of us have a roasting pan in their kitchen, so roasting your bones before boiling them is definitely not a problem. Another tool that is imperative to use for bone broth is a fine metal sieve. If you don't have one already, you can purchase a sieve that is large enough, as you don't want to spend one hour only for straining your broth little by little. What can you use for removing the meat from the bones? You can easily do this by using a slotted spoon or tongs. How should you actually separate it all and end up with your broth? Place the meat and the bones in a separate recipient and strain the broth in a large bowl. Afterwards you can ladle it into mason jars whose mouth is large enough. Store everything in the fridge if you plan to consume the broth within one week. If you want to freeze some of your broth, you can also use plastic recipients if they are better fit for your freezer. Alternatively you can use ice cubes trays if you want to defreeze your broth quickly when you consume it.

What is next? How should you consume your bone broth? Should you eat it or drink it? Actually you can do both. Many people use it as a base for further more elaborate dishes (e.g. soups), which is certainly recommended. However you should only do this if you simultaneously save enough broth you can drink as such. Pretend it's tea or just use a cup and drink it as your daily detox medicine! You don't have to pour your broth in a soup plate or bowl, because it's just liquid and you will find it easier and more enjoyable to consume it as a drink that is both energizing and appetite-quenching.

4. The Best Bone Broth Recipes

Before introducing you to a few of the greatest recipes you can use to prepare your bone broth, you should know some general details about the duration and the method you can use for this purpose. You probably didn't like the idea of having to let the bones boil for hours. Well, of course it's more fun when your food is ready in less than an hour. However remember everything about cooking bone broth is worth the time, because so many precious nutrients will be slowly released into the liquid and in the end into your own body. It won't actually cost you much effort – it is only the duration of the cooking that may scare you a bit. So how are you going to deal with that? Can you literally go around doing your own business while your broth is boiling? Are you going to resort to magic tricks and "call" some witches to turn all this process into an intriguing scene from *Macbeth*?

Actually you don't have to. You will be able to manage your bone broth on your own. Right after you wake up, you should place the bones you choose for your broth in cold water while also adding some vinegar (or other acid to your liking). Just fill a pot with cold water and leave the bones there as you get ready for work, if you have to leave home at that hour. When you're almost ready to leave after 30-60 minutes, you can bring everything to a simmer. Remember to skim the liquid after you bring it to a boil. Don't worry, nothing will happen if you place enough water in the pot and you follow the rest of the instructions. Everything has to boil slowly and when you return from work you'll already have your broth. After you come back home, remove your broth pot from the stove, let it cool, and then remove the bones from the liquid. The broth has to be strained before you store it or consume it immediately. As explained earlier, you can even leave the pot on the stove for a longer time. Just keep in mind 8-10 hours is quite enough for a sufficient quantity of minerals and other nutrients to be released into the liquid.

• We will start with a simple, but very effective recipe for bone broth that is generally enough if you want to prepare tasty and healthy broth. All you need are the following ingredients:

- bones : 3-4 pounds or more (make sure you find a healthy source)
- 2-3 chicken feet (for extra gelatin)
- 1-2 onions
- 2-3 carrots
- 2 celery stalks

- 2 tablespoons of vinegar/lemon juice (alternatively you can use half a glass to one full glass of white or red wine)
- 1 bunch of parsley
- 1-2 tablespoons of salt
- 1 teaspoon peppercorns
- 3-4 cloves of garlic
- spices and herbs you like (e.g. dill, allspice, or rosemary)

Is this recipe difficult? Not at all. Start with getting quality bones. Ideally you should roast them if you buy them fresh. Some people use the carcass from the roast chicken they prepare (for an amazing taste). The rule of thumb is using 2 pounds of bones for one gallon of water. If you have several chicken carcasses and you want to keep your broth limited to one type of bones only, feel free to use how many you want! Otherwise purchase beef or turkey bones and roast them for exquisite taste. You only have to place them in a pan and roast them for about 30 minutes before throwing them in cold water and acid.

You should use a pot that is large enough for all the ingredients. For instance, find a minimum 5-gallon pot and let your bones soak in acid cold water for 30-60 minutes. Chop the vegetables and add them into the pot, then bring everything to a boil. Let the liquid reach a vigorous boil, then reduce everything to simmer and take your time. As explained before, it's good enough if you let your bone broth simmer for

8-10 hours. However do consider expanding the duration of the simmer, should you have lots of time. If you don't have to leave home for days and go on vacation, you can definitely leave the pot on the stove in a slow simmer for up to 24 hours. Fish bones usually need a shorter cooking time, while beef or pork can even stay on the stove for over 24 hours. During the first stages of simmer, you should check the pot and remove any impurities that surface. High quality bones (e.g. organic or grass-fed) will produce less foam. Add garlic and spices during the last half an hour of simmer. Take your pot off the stove and remove the bones from the broth. Use a metal strainer to get a pure liquid out of the whole thing. When it's cool enough, store the broth in glass jars in the fridge or freeze if you don't consume it within 6-7 days.

- Another recipe you can use adds some more vegetables and herbs to your broth in order to ensure a rare taste. Use the following ingredients:

- 3-4 kg bones (chicken carcasses, beef bones, lamb bones, turkey etc.)
- lemon juice or vinegar
- 2-3 carrots, 2-3 parsley roots, 2-3 celery stalks
- 1-2 onions and 1-2 leeks
- one tablespoon black peppercorns
- 4 handfulls of greens (lettuce, nettles, kale, chard, cavalo negro etc.)
- 1 big pinch of salt
- 1 big pinch of winter herbs (thyme, sage, rosemary)
- 1 bunch of parsley leaves

Apply all the cooking techniques you're already learned and bring everything to a simmer. If you use chicken carcasses which are still "fleshy" and not what has remained from other dishes, you can pull off the meat after about 30 minutes. Fresh chicken carcasses can be thus used for more than one purpose. Keep the bones boiling for what your consider to be your ideal time (remember you can leave chicken bones in a simmer for up to 12 hours and beef or lamb bones even for 48 hours). Add vegetables when it all starts simmering, but don't place any greens in the pot that soon. Only add them when your broth is almost ready. Herbs should be the last ingredients you place in your simmering pot. You will get a unique taste for your broth, no matter how many bone types you use. This broth tastes great even if you don't roast your bones before boiling them.

● Our next recipe is based on one type of bones only. You can prepare an incredibly tasty beef bone broth if you use the following ingredients:

- 3-4 kg beef bones (from your local farmer or a quality supermarket/butcher's)
- 2-3 carrots, 2-3 parsley roots
- 1 large can of green peas
- 1-2 onions
- 7 smashed garlic cloves
- 2-3 bay leaves
- 2 tablespoons vinegar or lemon juice (alternatively one glass of red wine would also be great)

- salt
- mushrooms (use how many you want, ideally up to half a kilo)

Beef bones are especially delicious when roasted before used for broth. Follow the steps you already know from the other recipes and bring everything to a simmer in a large pot. Don't forget to let the bones soak in cold water in which you poured acid and also placed the bay leaves. Add vegetables and peas together with the bones in the beginning. Mushrooms should be placed in the pot a bit later, in the last hour of simmering. Add smashed garlic in the end, when you have less than half an hour left. If you're short on time, leave the pot on the stove for 8-10 hours. Separate the solid ingredients from the broth by means of a strainer. Drink the liquid as such after it cools a bit or store it in a glass container. If you use fatty bones, remember to remove the fat from the surface of the broth after you leave it in the fridge. It will definitely taste better. Enjoy!

• If you love the highly nourishing Shiitake mushrooms, you will also adore our next recipe. They are extremely valued in Asia where they are considered to be a symbol of longevity. Most people consume them not only for the great taste, but also for their health-supporting properties. Shiitake mushrooms are known to improve the cardiovascular system, to boost the immune system, and to provide you with a highly valuable and natural source of iron and amino acids. So what do you need for this special bone broth apart from Shiitake mushrooms? Here are the ingredients:

- 3-4 kg beef, pork, or veal bones (if you can easily find and afford veal, don't hesitate)
- Shiitake mushrooms (up to half of kilo)
- 2-3 carrots, 2-3 celery stalks, 2 parsnip roots
- 2 onions
- bacon (a few slices)
- kombu (Japanese seaweed)
- 2 bay leaves
- vinegar or wine
- herbs (sage, parsley, thyme, or rosemary)

For this recipe you should roast the vegetables together with the bones before you place them all in cold water. Pour your acid in water (wine or vinegar would be great for this recipe). Just as in our previous recipes, bring everything to simmer and remove impurities. Bacon should be added in the beginning together with the bones and vegetables. Place the kombu kelp in the same water for an extremely savory flavor. Add mushrooms later in the broth, after it has simmered for at least 8 hours. Regulate taste with any herbs of your choice and use a sieve to separate the liquid from everything else. As you can see, this recipe is distinctively Asian and it offers you many nutrients together with a unique taste.

• In the end of this chapter we will show you how to prepare delicious chicken bone broth in a few simple steps. As a basis you should use the carcasses from your roasted chicken dish. The taste will be lacking if you choose fresh bones for this recipe.

Ingredients:

- 3 roast chicken carcasses (alternatively you can use 1-2 roast turkey carcasses)
- 2-3 carrots, 2-3 parsley roots, 2-3 celery roots
- 4 potatoes
- 2 red peppers
- 2-3 tomatoes
- 2 beet roots (optional …for a smashing additional taste and some more color)
- 2-3 bay leaves
- 2 onions or leeks
- ginger root (a few slices)
- 1 bunch of parsley leaves
- salt and pepper
- 2 tablespoons of vinegar or lemon juice (alternatively white wine is great for these ingredients)
- herbs to your discretion (basil, sage, allspice, and estragon are delicious for this recipe)

Place your roast chicken carcasses in cold water in which you also added acid, bay leaves, and vegetables. You can leave the tomatoes for a later moment, but make sure you add the rest from the beginning. Bring the pot to simmer and remove impurities. This recipe works quite well if you keep the bones boiling for 8-10 hours. Remove the solid parts from the broth and sieve the liquid. Consume immediately or store in the fridge after it cools. You will get a terrific taste!

As you could see from our recipe recommendations, you can adjust the simmering time. If you don't care about time and having some really tasty and nutritionally dense broth is more important to you, go for the 24-48 hours version. You can leave the pot on the stove as you sleep. Place your bones (and optionally meat) in water and add acid of your choice. Bring everything to a boil after you let the bones soak in acid liquid. Add vegetables and skim the broth. Reduce heat and let the pot simmer. You can leave fish bones simmer for 5-24 hours, chicken bones for 8-12 hours, and lamb, pork, or beef bones for 12-48 hours. Herbs should always be added later. Most people throw vegetables in the broth right from the start, but this is actually a matter of choice. If you prefer a fresher taste, you can add them later, during the last 1-2 hours of simmering. After you remove the bones and meat and you sieve the broth, you can keep everything in the fridge for up to 7 days and in the freezer for up to 6 months. Of course serving some broth immediately is highly recommended and you'll probably hardly be able to resist the smell and taste while you separate your broth.

5. Is Bone Broth a Magic Potion for Your Health? The Great Benefits of Bone Broth

After hearing so much about this powerful food, you must be wondering what makes it so special and why there are more and more people nowadays who include it in their eating habits. Is there a bone broth trend? The answer is complex and it starts from the fact that this food is great to use in a broader program like the paleo diet. Many people have consumed it intensively and they have noticed an incredible improvement in their health. For this reason they shared their "secret" with others. It is true that bone broth is one of the most sought after types of food nowadays. There's an interesting paradox about bone broth: one the one hand, this food is very old, but we have forgotten what kept our ancestors healthy with so much junk food bombarding us on every corner; on the other hand, people who focus on healthy and natural nutrition rediscovered the value of bone broth and started "promoting" this wonderful food.

Since many people talk about its benefits and bone broth is after all a quite simple food type, maybe you are a bit skeptical about its properties and about what it can do for you. Why does everyone talk about it as if it were a magic potion? Should you really trust those who praise it or is it just something "in fashion" that many have blindly adopted? While nobody is trying to convince you that you'll live eternally if you consume bone broth, there are definitely significant benefits to your health once you include this food in your daily routines. Let's see what bone broth can heal and who should intensively consume it.

First of all, there's a very simple truth we often ignore: we should eat things that contain the same substances as the parts of the body we want to treat or heal. It makes sense scientifically, doesn't it? Thus it is only natural that bone broth will have important effects on the health of your bones and teeth. The high amount of minerals in animal bones will directly feed your own bone structure and you won't have to resort to myriad supplements to keep your bones healthy. People who are older should start consuming bone broth right away! If you have osteoporosis, joint pain, rheumatism, or arthritis, don't waste any more time and start consuming bone broth, because the nourishing substances in bones, skin, and ligaments will improve the condition of your body. Bone broth will alleviate your symptoms after a while, provided that you consume this magic food regularly.

What is the secret of bone broth? You may think it sounds so much like ambrosia. "Is that what gods eat to stay cool?" you may wonder. Actually the force of bone broth lies in its multifaceted benefits. You can use it for your immune system, for your bones, and also for your energy levels. Ultimately through its multiple amazing effects bone broth can bring back your morning wood!

So it is like a drink of the gods after all. It doesn't have aphrodisiac properties as such, at least not in an immediate way. If you consume ginger, oysters, or royal jelly, your sexual desire as well as your prowess will visibly improve. You will get an energy boost right away! This is probably something most of us know and have already included in our lives. What many of us don't know is that bone broth can lead to similar results in quite a different way. Bone broth acts more slowly and subtly on your organism, but rest assured that after you consume it on a daily basis for longer periods, you will sense a clear improvement in your overall health. If you are young, you are of course welcome to keep your energy levels very high. However bone broth is especially recommendable to people who are not in their 20s anymore. If you are in your 40s and older, your health needs support more than ever. Besides, you will want to keep your sexuality (and your sexual performance) on a satisfactory level even if you grow older. Nothing works better than bone broth for this purpose in the long run!

Bone broth is a priceless source of minerals that you can ingest in a form your body can easily absorb. There is a high quantity of calcium, magnesium, silicon, phosphorus, gelatin, collagen, glucosamine, sulfur chlondroitin etc. in bones. Your regular food doesn't usually contain enough of such substances for your whole body and most of us resort to supplements to keep their levels balanced. Instead of spending money on vitamins and minerals, why shouldn't you consume bone broth on a daily basis? It's worth more than one capsule or tablet of your usual multivitamins and it also tastes great. Besides, you can eat or drink as much bone broth as you want, there's no limit to this magic food in a day. Absolutely no side effects! You will only bring your body more energy and you'll get it used to extracting its nutrients in the most natural way possible.

Bone broth is extraordinary if you have to fight some illness and recover fast. For instance, it will help you get better in a much shorter time when you catch a cold or the flu, when you have a sore throat, when you have a mild infection in your lungs or sinuses etc. Of course, if you suffer from more severe inflammation, infection, or viruses, you should not limit yourself to consuming bone broth. Always follow the treatment prescribed by your medical specialist.

However bone broth is great additional medicine for basically any kind of ailment you may be affected by. When it comes to something as simple as a cold or the flu, you are actually very likely to be cured quickly only by eating a lot of broth. Why do you think our parents or grandparents used to feed us with chicken soup when we were sick? The scientific answer is that chicken contains cysteine, a natural amino acid that can make the mucus in your lungs thinner and thus help you expel it. Anything that affects your mouth, lungs, throat, or nose will go away faster if you eat chicken bone broth. Keep in mind chicken soup is also good for such sickness, but nothing will be as potent as the broth in which the bones have released all their high amounts of minerals and nutrients for hours in a row.

Bone broth is like a balm for your gut. As Dr. Alejandro Junger explains in his book *Clean Gut*, our overall health depends on how well our digestive system functions. When there is an imbalance in your gut, your whole body suffers, although you may not realize the root cause is in your belly. You should know that bone broth has amazingly positive effects on your whole gut, since it contains many substances that facilitate the production of gastro-intestinal juices which play an important part in breaking down your food into nutrients. The gelatin contained by the bone broth attracts and holds liquids (including your gastric juices) and thus it supports your overall digestion and metabolism. Many digestive ailments can be cured by means of bone broth: a leaking gut, ulcer, flatulence, irritable bowel syndrome etc. Bone broth soothes your gut lining and at the same time it regulates the production of gastric juices, thus improving your overall digestion.

Bone broth can help you combat any kind of infection you may have in your body or you may be prone to developing. If your immune system is not as strong as it should be or if you are getting older, just add this wonder food to your daily menu. It will be like topping your life with a few years more. If you have any kind of inflammation (around your eyes, in your teeth, in your lungs, your gall bladder, your reproductive system etc.), bone broth will facilitate healing. Bones contain amino acids such as glycine, proline, and arginine which are well-known for their anti-inflammatory effects. Bone broth can help you cure joint inflammation, muscle tension, and even something as severe as sepsis (an inflammation that is spread in the whole organism). Drink plenty of broth every day and you'll see that any treatment prescribed by your doctor is enhanced!

Each of the three amino acids mentioned above play a major role in your health. Glycine is the substance that prevents breakdown of protein tissue (e.g. muscle). It also acts as an antioxidant and it facilitates detoxification processes in our organism. Apart from these effects it has directly on the tissue of your body, it is an important neurotransmitter that regulates sleep and other mental processes. A higher amount of glycine in your body will improve your memory, mood, and sleep patterns. Glycine also regulates sugar levels in your blood and it improves the quality of your muscles by means of keratin. Proline is the substance that lies at the root of joint, gut, and skin health. It helps your cartilages regenerate, it supports your digestive system, and it plays a major part in combating cellulite. Proline also helps in treating arterosclerosis, since it leads to a release of cholesterol buildup in your blood. Your circulatory system will benefit a lot if you consume bone broth. Arginine acts like a magic balm on your immune system as well as on your liver. If you eat food that is rich in arginine, your immunity will get a notable boost, your growth will be facilitated (if you are a kid, for instance), and any damaged cells in your liver will be regenerated. Last, but not least, arginine acts like a catalyst for sperm production, which brings us to one of the most powerful benefits of bone broth, namely enhanced sexual performance, energy, and prowess.

Besides acting directly on the health of your bones, this magic food contains so many minerals and vitamins that will automatically improve the condition of your hair and skin, too. Did you know collagen is what keeps your skin firm, elastic, and young? Well, you'll hardly ever find any food that contains more collagen than bone broth, especially if you also use plenty of ligaments and skin when you prepare it. Most people have to purchase a special facial cream or apply collagen directly on their skin and lines. They pay a lot of money for a good cosmetic product that includes this essential substance for their skin whose quantity in our organism actually decreases as we grow older. It would be mere insanity to ignore such a valuable natural source of collagen as bone broth, don't you think so? However it would be wrong to think that collagen is only necessary for skin health. This substance protects gastric lining and a higher quantity of collagen in your digestive system and your whole body will alleviate ulcer, chron's, colitis, and gastro-intestinal reflux. Gelatin and collagen are also immensely curative and important in combating cellulite. It improves skin quality and elasticity. The skin that covers your whole body will stay supple. Just picture that now you only have to drink lots of bone broth instead of buying anti-wrinkle cream or anti-cellulite gel that has to be applied on each affected area! If you consume bone broth instead of coke or beer, you will save your body the discomfort of receiving useless and harmful additives. Instead you will nourish your body and skin with minerals and other essential substances that help your skin regenerate and stay firm. Moreover, your hair and your nails will also benefit from all the nutrients contained in bone broth. If you consume this food regularly, you will notice your hair grows more shiny and more healthy and your nails are spotless and tough.

Your metabolism will be improved by means of bone broth, because bones contain a high quantity of glutamine. This substance acts as some sort of metabolic fuel for your gut (especially for cells in your small intestine). Additionally glutamine is great medicine for muscle building. If you think you are losing muscle because of the aging process or because you have got thinner, all you have to do is consume a lot of bone broth.

Given its high detoxification potential, bone broth can be used as an essential ingredient in a fast or another kind of detox program. Many people use natural juice or a cleanser prepared by mixing maple syrup, hot pepper, and lemon juice. While we are not necessarily challenging the strong detox effects of such a Master Cleanser which can also help people lose unwanted weight, you have to be informed that bone broth is a remarkable alternative to it. Other people use yogurt or green tea for detox purposes. The bottom line is that nothing contains as many nutrients as bone broth. If you are interested in a detox diet or you have tried intermittent fasting, you should consider using bone broth as your basic detox drink by all means. It will help your organism stay nourished during your detox/fast which can last from days to weeks, depending on how harsh you want it to be. The longer you fast on water or liquids only, the more dangerous it is for your organism from specific points of view. While we agree with the value of fasting for cell regeneration, we cannot ignore the fact that having to feed on tea or juice only for days in a row can weaken your organism and even your performance at work. Bone broth is highly concentrated and nourishing and you risk much less if you base your fast on this "cleanse". Your detoxification will have a powerful weapon, while your body will still get its nutrients from such a rich source of minerals and proteins as bones. Moreover, by consuming a nicely prepared bone broth which also tastes appealing, you can appease your hunger or your craving for something delicious during your detox program.

Last, but not least, bone broth is great fuel for your brain cells. Not only does it boost your immune system and your overall energy levels, but also it enhances memory and intellectual capacity as well as performance. It's great to have your bone broth supplies even if you're a kid or a student and you have to pass your exams. Bone broth helps your mood stay positive and bright. It is also great medicine when you have to struggle with stress or depression. Your whole nervous system is supported by means of bone broth. It goes without saying that adults should definitely turn this food into their "daily bread" if they want to stay one step ahead of natural aging processes. You can start when you're in your 30s and you will certainly not regret it in your 40s or 50s. Drink as much bone broth as you can and do it regularly, if you want evident effects.

6. Bonus Tips and Tricks

How can you make the most out of your bone broth? Are there extra "tricks" that you can use to increase the nourishing potential of your broth or to allow for a series of variations once you include it in your routines?

• You can add more than chicken legs to your broth regardless of the types of bones you use. Chicken heads, necks, and wings will increase the concentration of minerals and collagen in your broth. Buying bones that are big enough to provide you with some marrow as well is also important. We are much too accustomed to consider only chicken breast or other kinds of meat with lots of muscle to be worth eating. They surely are, but for your special bone broth don't throw away anything. On the contrary, you can purchase chicken heads, legs, knuckles, sternum, vertebrae, or necks separately from the butcher's to enrich your broth. By using all the parts of an animal's body in your broth, you will incorporate all the nutrients and benefits you usually discard due to living in a time and a culture that appreciates only the softer and "meaty" parts for their solidity. Keep in mind you can combine bone types except for fish. Cook fish alone, or else you'll get an unpleasant jungle of tastes. When you use fish, never throw away the fish heads, although it may seem a bit gross to place them in your pot. Ignore anything you're used to for the sake of having even more beneficial substances in your broth – you won't eat them as such, after all. What kind of fish should you use? Avoid using oily fish such as salmon ... although it was probably not your first choice for bone broth. The optimal ideas for fish bone broth are rockfish or snapper.

• Should you use meat together with your bones? The answer is yes, because this way you'll benefit both from the minerals in bones and from the high amount of proteins in meat. You'll just double your nutrients! Of course, you can leave some of the "good meat" for 1-2 hours only and then use it for the preparation of another dish. For extra flavor add fresh meat. It can also have enough skin, as this part of the animal body is also quite rich in nutrients. Avoid placing a lot of fat in your broth, because you'll affect the taste negatively and you may feel a bit sick when you drink it. You will also do better without any fat that you can gather and remove with a spoon after your broth stays in the fridge for a while.

• For enhanced nourishing qualities, you can add astragalus or kombu. The former is the root of a herb that is widely used in Chinese cuisine and medicine.

If you can find and purchase it easily, add this ingredient for a stronger boost of your immune system. The latter is a Japanese basis for stock and soups. This brown kelp has high mineral content and it also adds to the taste.

• Some people have discovered that adding eggshells in the broth can be beneficial, although it does nothing when it comes to taste. Since egg shells are an important source of calcium as well as of other great substances such as collagen, glucosamine, or hyaluronic acid, why shouldn't you take advantage of their properties? We never consume egg shells and, if you have to find a method to include their nourishing substances in your diet without having to actually eat the shells, what could be better than placing them in your broth pot?

• Can you use a pressure cooker? Ideally not. You will lose more than half of the benefits of bone broth. This magic food is meant to be cooked slowly to guarantee the release of every bit of nutrient in liquid. If you are in a hurry once or twice, you can of course also resort to your pressure cooker, but don't make it your regular pot! Keep your patience under control and don't spoil the broth through a bad decision of one single cook.

• If you buy larger bones, you could chop them to ensure a better and faster transition of the nutrients in water. This way you'll shorten the duration of broth preparation to some extent. However never throw any bit of marrow away! That's likely the most precious part of the bones that will feed your body so generously.

7. How to Add Flavor to Your Bone Broth

It is quite important to roast your bones before simmering if taste is your priority. You have nothing to lose in terms of nutrients, so why not? Feel free to turn your broth into an unforgettable dish. Fish bones can work better fresh. Other types of bones definitely have better flavor when roasted. If you like the taste a lot, roast your vegetables, too.

Use any kinds of vegetables, greens, and herbs. Nothing is forbidden …just remember to be a bit more intransigent when it comes to cabbage, broccoli, and cauliflower. For a more attractive taste you can add asparagus, zucchini, kale, nettles, spinach, capers, artichoke, endives, watercress, turnips etc. How about legumes? You don't really need them for taste, unless you love the flavor of roast beef and beans. You can try diversifying your routine after you're already an expert in bone broth…but keep in mind adding peas, beans, or lentils might also make your broth harder to tolerate (e.g. such ingredients are known to cause flatulence). If you add more rare and delicious vegetables or greens, you might want to consider not leaving them in the broth till they "melt," unless you want to use them all for purée.

For extra taste you can always add garlic, ginger, leek, vine leafs, olives etc. Additionally you can pour 1-2 tablespoons of olive oil in your broth or alternatively use a lump of butter for better taste. You are free to use spices at will, no matter how hot: pepper, allspice, thyme, basil, chili powder, estragon, rosemary, anis, majoran, dill etc. Just don't mix too many, if you don't already know their taste harmonizes well. For instance, placing estragon and basil in the same dish may be futile and not recommended, since such herbs have a distinctive flavor of their own that should be the basis for a certain dish. Eggplant, pumpkin, or avocado can make for an exotic and interesting taste. Combine them with chicken or turkey bones only. Avoid "heavy" spices such as curry, cardamom, mustard, or cumin.

Replacing your vinegar with wine is a great tip for extra taste, especially when you use fish, venison, or chicken bones. Naturally you should stick to the rule of thumb of using white wine for white meat and red wine for the rest. Experiment with the taste first, because not everyone prefers wine to lemon juice or vinegar when they have to drink plenty of broth during one day. Lemon juice may be the best solution to make the liquid highly tolerable for your stomach in large quantities.

For a stronger and more rapid effect on your overall health, but first and foremost on your energy levels and your sexual life, always include other well-known "powerhouse food" in your bone broth. Add ginseng, garlic, asparagus, celery, spinach, kale, hot peppers, yohimbe, and slices of ginger (or powder) in your broth. Of course, you won't be able to include every revitalizing and aphrodisiac ingredient you know, lest you negatively affect the taste. Bone broth with honey or chocolate sounds scary and repelling, doesn't it? Well, what you can do is add anything that tastes a bit sour, bitter, or spicy. Anything else is welcome as long as it has some mixed, subtle, and delicious taste which is not sweet.

8. Conclusions

In this book we introduced you to the myriad benefits of a seemingly simple and tasteless food that some of us only use once in a while as a basis for more sophisticated dishes. It is essential that you understand this food was widely used by our ancestors. We have forgotten how to take advantage of everything that nature (both animal and vegetal) can offer us. We are mainly interested in delicatessen, technology, and luxury nowadays. This beginner's guide to the benefits of bone broth has showed you not only why it is so important to rediscover this magic food and include it in your diet, but also how you can best prepare it to get an unforgettable taste as well. Nobody is trying to convince you to drink something that tastes unpleasant all day long, although some detox programs or some harsher medical diets may imply that as well. In our guide we aimed at helping you turn bone broth into a dish that is absolutely worth including in your daily menu. You don't have to consume it out of obligation. Now you know how to squeeze everything it has to offer by enriching the taste of bones.

You are now probably already convinced that you only have a lot to gain if you start consuming bone broth. This is your new treatment for many ailments, from purely physical ones to mental deregulations or undesirable phenomena. Not only will you get an energy boost, but also you'll have better memory, a more positive mood, and enhanced beauty. Your immune system, your gut, your skin, and your sexuality …they will all benefit after you start your bone broth program. Your overall levels of energy will be higher, aging processes are kept at bay for a longer while, and bone broth directly influences the activity of certain sexual glands. Thus it would not be far-fetched at all to say bone broth will bring your back your youth and vigor. Your sexual life will be visibly improved by means of bone broth. That said in case you are not exactly young anymore, you can now use bone broth for getting back your morning wood. It works!

Made in the USA
Lexington, KY
15 May 2016